Chair Yoga Awesome Guide for Beginners

Incorporating Chair Yoga into Your Routine

By

Eamon Craig

Copyright@2024

Table of Contents

CHAPTER 1

Introduction

1.1 What is Chair Yoga?

Chair yoga is a modified form of yoga that is specifically designed to be practiced while sitting on a chair or using a chair for support. It incorporates gentle stretches, breathing exercises, and meditation techniques, making it accessible to individuals of all ages and fitness levels, including those with mobility issues or physical limitations.

Unlike traditional yoga practices that often require getting up and down from the floor or holding challenging standing poses, chair yoga offers a safe and supportive way to experience the benefits of yoga while remaining seated. It focuses on improving flexibility, strength, balance, and relaxation, all within the comfort and stability of a chair.

The practice of chair yoga typically involves a series of gentle movements and stretches that target different parts of the body, such as the neck, shoulders, spine, hips, and legs. These movements are adapted from traditional yoga poses and can be easily modified to accommodate individual needs and abilities.

Chair yoga also emphasizes mindful breathing techniques and relaxation exercises to help calm the mind, reduce stress, and promote overall well-being. By incorporating mindfulness and meditation practices, chair yoga encourages practitioners to cultivate awareness of their breath, body, and thoughts, fostering a deeper sense of inner peace and tranquility.

One of the key advantages of chair yoga is its versatility and accessibility. It can be practiced virtually anywhere – at home, in the office, or even while traveling – with minimal space and equipment required. All that is needed is a sturdy chair and a willingness to explore gentle movement and breathwork.

chair yoga offers a gentle yet effective way to experience the numerous benefits of yoga, regardless of age, fitness level, or physical ability. It provides a supportive environment for individuals to improve their overall health and well-being, enhance their flexibility and strength, and find greater ease and relaxation in both body and mind.

1.2 Benefits of Chair Yoga

Chair yoga offers a wide range of benefits for both physical and mental well-being, making it an ideal practice

for individuals of all ages and abilities.
Some of the key benefits of chair yoga
include:

1. Improved Flexibility: Chair yoga
    incorporates gentle stretches and
    movements that help to increase
    flexibility and range of motion in
    the muscles and joints. Regular
    practice can help to alleviate
    stiffness and tension, promoting
    greater ease of movement and
    comfort.

2. Enhanced Strength: Despite being
    seated, chair yoga poses can still
    engage and strengthen various
    muscle groups, including the core,
    arms, legs, and back. Over time,
    this can lead to improved muscle
    tone, stability, and overall
    strength.

3. Better Posture: Chair yoga
    promotes awareness of body
    alignment and encourages proper

posture while sitting. By
strengthening the muscles that
support the spine and improving
alignment, chair yoga can help to
reduce slouching and alleviate
back pain.

4. Increased Balance and Stability:
   Chair yoga poses often
   incorporate elements of balance
   and stability, which can help to
   improve proprioception and
   coordination. Practicing balance
   poses while seated on a chair can
   enhance stability and reduce the
   risk of falls, particularly for older
   adults.

5. Stress Reduction: Chair yoga
   emphasizes mindfulness and
   relaxation techniques, such as
   deep breathing and meditation,
   which can help to calm the
   nervous system and reduce stress
   levels. Regular practice can
   promote a sense of peace,

tranquility, and overall emotional well-being.

6. Pain Management: Chair yoga can be beneficial for individuals dealing with chronic pain conditions, such as arthritis, fibromyalgia, or lower back pain. Gentle stretches and movements can help to alleviate tension, improve circulation, and reduce pain and discomfort.

7. Improved Circulation: The gentle movements and stretches practiced in chair yoga can help to stimulate blood flow and circulation throughout the body. This can promote better oxygenation of tissues, improve cardiovascular health, and reduce the risk of circulation-related issues.

8. Enhanced Mood and Mental Clarity: Chair yoga encourages

mindfulness and present moment awareness, which can help to reduce feelings of anxiety, depression, and mental fatigue. Practicing chair yoga regularly can promote a sense of inner calm, clarity, and emotional balance.

9. Accessibility and Inclusivity: One of the greatest benefits of chair yoga is its accessibility to individuals with limited mobility, injuries, or disabilities. By adapting traditional yoga poses to be performed while seated, chair yoga ensures that everyone can experience the benefits of yoga, regardless of physical ability.

Chair yoga offers a gentle yet effective way to improve flexibility, strength, balance, and overall well-being. Whether you're dealing with physical limitations, seeking stress relief, or simply looking to incorporate more movement into your day, chair yoga provides a versatile and accessible practice that can be enjoyed by all.

CHAPTER 2

Getting Started

2.1 Setting Up Your Space

Before you begin practicing chair yoga, it's important to create a comfortable and safe environment that supports your practice. Here are some tips for setting up your space:

1. Find a Quiet and Clutter-Free Area: Choose a quiet and clutter-free area where you can focus without distractions. Clear away any furniture or objects that may obstruct your movement or cause accidents.

2. Use a Sturdy Chair: Select a sturdy chair without wheels that provides stable support. Avoid chairs with armrests that are too high, as they may restrict your

movement during certain poses. Ensure that the chair is placed on a flat surface to prevent tipping or sliding.

3. Position Your Chair: Place your chair on a non-slip surface, such as a yoga mat or carpet, to prevent it from sliding. Position the chair so that you have enough space to extend your arms and legs comfortably in all directions.

4. Create a Comfortable Seating Arrangement: Situate yourself in the center of the chair with your feet flat on the ground and your knees aligned with your hips. Adjust the height of the chair if necessary to maintain a neutral spine and avoid slouching.

5. Gather Props and Accessories: Depending on your needs and preferences, you may want to gather props and accessories to

enhance your practice. This may include a yoga strap, yoga blocks, or a folded blanket for added support and comfort.

6. Set the Mood: Create a calming atmosphere by dimming the lights, playing soft music, or lighting candles or incense. Engage your senses to create a peaceful and inviting space for your practice.

7. Dress Comfortably: Wear loose, comfortable clothing that allows for unrestricted movement. Avoid tight or constricting clothing that may restrict your breathing or circulation during practice.

8. Stay Hydrated: Have a bottle of water nearby to stay hydrated throughout your practice. Taking regular sips of water can help to replenish fluids lost through

sweating and keep you feeling energized and focused.

Setting up your space thoughtfully and mindfully, you can create an environment that supports and enhances your chair yoga practice. Remember to listen to your body and make any necessary adjustments to ensure your comfort and safety throughout your practice.

2.2 Choosing the Right Chair

Selecting the right chair is essential for a safe and effective chair yoga practice. Here are some factors to consider when choosing the chair that best suits your needs:

1. Stability: Choose a chair that is stable and sturdy, with a solid frame and supportive structure. Avoid chairs that wobble or feel

flimsy, as they may compromise your balance and safety during practice.

2. Seat Height: Opt for a chair with a seat height that allows your feet to rest comfortably flat on the ground with your knees bent at a 90-degree angle. This ensures proper alignment and support for your spine and pelvis.

3. Seat Width and Depth: Look for a chair with a seat that is wide and deep enough to accommodate your body comfortably. Avoid chairs with seats that are too narrow or shallow, as they may cause discomfort or restrict your movement.

4. Back Support: Choose a chair with adequate back support to maintain proper spinal alignment during practice. Look for chairs with a straight backrest or

adjustable lumbar support to
minimize strain on your back and
neck.

5. Armrests: Consider whether you
    prefer a chair with or without
    armrests based on your personal
    comfort and mobility needs.
    Armrests can provide additional
    support and stability during
    certain poses, but they may also
    limit your range of motion in
    others.

6. Material and Cushioning: Select a
    chair with comfortable cushioning
    and breathable upholstery to
    enhance your comfort during
    practice. Avoid chairs with overly
    soft or plush seats, as they may
    make it difficult to maintain
    stability and alignment.

7. Portability: If you plan to practice
    chair yoga in different locations
    or while traveling, choose a

lightweight and portable chair that is easy to transport. Look for chairs that fold or stack compactly for convenient storage and mobility.

8. Personal Preferences: Ultimately, the best chair for your chair yoga practice is one that meets your individual preferences and needs. Take the time to test out different chairs and consider factors such as aesthetics, durability, and ease of maintenance before making your final decision.

Choosing the right chair for your chair yoga practice, you can create a supportive and comfortable environment that enhances your overall experience and enjoyment. Experiment with different chairs until you find the one that feels most comfortable and supportive for your body and practice.

2.3 Clothing and Equipment

Choosing the appropriate clothing and equipment for chair yoga can enhance your comfort and ease during practice. Here are some considerations to keep in mind:

1. Comfortable Clothing: Select loose-fitting, breathable clothing that allows for unrestricted movement. Avoid tight or constricting garments that may restrict your range of motion or cause discomfort during practice. Opt for lightweight materials such as cotton or moisture-wicking fabrics to help keep you cool and dry.

2. Layers: Consider wearing layers that can be easily added or removed as needed to regulate your body temperature during practice. This allows you to adjust to changes in room temperature or

your level of exertion without interrupting your practice.

3. Supportive Footwear: While chair yoga is primarily practiced while seated, supportive footwear can still play a role in your comfort and stability. Choose shoes with good arch support and non-slip soles to provide traction and stability when standing or transitioning between poses.

4. Accessories: Depending on your preferences and needs, you may want to incorporate accessories to enhance your practice. This may include:

   - Yoga Props: Consider using props such as yoga blocks, straps, or blankets to modify poses and provide additional support or stability as needed.

- Cushions or Pillows: If you have discomfort or pressure points while sitting, use cushions or pillows to provide extra padding and support for your back, hips, or knees.

- Water Bottle: Stay hydrated throughout your practice by having a water bottle nearby. Sipping water regularly can help replenish fluids lost through sweating and keep you feeling refreshed and energized.

5. Jewelry and Accessories: Remove any jewelry or accessories that may interfere with your practice or cause discomfort during movement. This includes watches, bracelets, rings, or necklaces that may catch on clothing or equipment.

6. Comfortable Hair Accessories: If you have long hair, consider using hair ties or clips to keep your hair away from your face and neck during practice. This can help prevent distractions and discomfort while moving through different poses.

7. Personal Hygiene: Practice good personal hygiene by wearing clean, comfortable clothing and avoiding strong scents or perfumes that may be distracting or bothersome to yourself or others in the class.

Choosing the right clothing and equipment for your chair yoga practice, you can create a comfortable and supportive environment that allows you to fully engage in your practice and experience its many benefits. Experiment with different options to find what works best for you and enhances your overall yoga experience.

CHAPTER 3

Basic Chair Yoga Poses

3.1 Seated Mountain Pose

Seated Mountain Pose, also known as "Tadasana," is a foundational yoga pose that promotes alignment, stability, and grounding. Here's how to practice it while seated in a chair:

- Sit comfortably on the edge of your chair with your feet flat on the ground and your spine tall.

- Place your hands on your thighs or knees, palms facing down.

- Press down through your sit bones to lengthen your spine, lifting your chest and gently drawing your shoulder blades together.

- Engage your core muscles to support your spine and maintain a neutral pelvis.

- Relax your shoulders away from your ears and soften your facial muscles.

- Close your eyes if comfortable, and take several deep breaths, focusing on grounding through your sit bones and lengthening through the crown of your head.

- Hold the pose for 30 seconds to 1 minute, continuing to breathe deeply and mindfully.

- To release, gently open your eyes and return to a neutral seated position.

Benefits: Seated Mountain Pose helps to improve posture, increase awareness of alignment, and promote a sense of grounding and stability.

3.2 Seated Forward Bend

Seated Forward Bend, or "Paschimottanasana," stretches the spine, hamstrings, and lower back, while also calming the mind and relieving stress. Here's how to practice it using a chair for support:

- Sit upright on the edge of your chair with your feet hip-width apart and your spine tall.

- Inhale as you reach your arms overhead, lengthening through your spine.

- Exhale and hinge forward from your hips, leading with your chest as you fold forward over your thighs.

- Keep your back flat and your neck long, avoiding rounding your spine or straining your neck.

- Place your hands on your shins,
  ankles, or the seat of the chair for
  support, depending on your
  flexibility.

- Relax your neck and shoulders,
  and breathe deeply into the
  stretch, feeling a gentle opening in
  your hamstrings and lower back.

- Hold the pose for 30 seconds to 1
  minute, continuing to breathe
  deeply and relax into the stretch.

- To release, inhale as you slowly
  lift your torso back up to a seated
  position, keeping your spine tall.

Benefits: Seated Forward Bend stretches
the spine, hamstrings, and lower back,
while also calming the mind and
relieving stress. It can help improve
flexibility, relieve tension in the back
and neck, and promote relaxation.

3.3 Seated Twist

Seated Twist, also known as "Ardha Matsyendrasana," is a gentle yoga pose that helps to increase spinal mobility, stretch the back muscles, and aid in digestion. Here's how to practice Seated Twist using a chair for support:

1. Sit comfortably on the edge of your chair with your feet flat on the ground and your spine tall.

2. Place your hands on your knees or thighs.

3. Inhale deeply, lengthening your spine.

4. Exhale and twist your torso to the right, using your hands on your knees or thighs to deepen the twist.

5. Keep your spine tall and your shoulders relaxed as you twist, avoiding any strain or discomfort.

6. Gaze over your right shoulder if comfortable, or keep your gaze forward.

7. Hold the twist for 15-30 seconds, breathing deeply and maintaining awareness of your breath.

8. Inhale to come back to the center, lengthening your spine.

9. Exhale and repeat the twist to the left side, following the same steps.

10. Hold the twist for 15-30 seconds, breathing deeply and maintaining awareness of your breath.

11. Inhale to come back to the center, lengthening your spine.

12. Repeat the seated twist sequence 2-3 times on each side, alternating between right and left.

Benefits:

- Seated Twist helps to increase spinal mobility and flexibility.

- It stretches the muscles along the spine, including the back, shoulders, and chest.

- The twisting motion can aid in digestion and improve circulation in the abdominal area.

- Seated Twist also promotes relaxation and can help to relieve tension and stiffness in the back and shoulders.

Caution:

- Avoid forcing the twist or overstretching. Listen to your body and only twist as far as feels comfortable.

- If you have any pre-existing spinal or back injuries, consult with a healthcare professional before practicing Seated Twist or any other yoga pose.

3.4 Seated Cat-Cow Stretch

The Seated Cat-Cow Stretch is a gentle yoga movement that helps to increase spinal mobility, release tension in the back, and improve posture. Here's how to practice it:

1. Sit comfortably on the edge of your chair with your feet flat on the ground and your spine tall.

2. Place your hands on your knees or thighs.

3. Inhale deeply as you arch your back and lift your chest forward, bringing your shoulder blades together (this is the "Cow" position).

4. Exhale slowly as you round your spine, tucking your chin towards

your chest and drawing your belly button towards your spine (this is the "Cat" position).

5. Continue to move fluidly between the Cat and Cow positions with your breath, inhaling as you arch into Cow and exhaling as you round into Cat.

6. Repeat this movement for 6-8 breaths, focusing on the fluidity of the motion and the stretch along your spine.

7. After your final exhale, return to a neutral seated position with your spine tall.

Benefits:

- The Seated Cat-Cow Stretch helps to improve spinal flexibility and mobility.

- It stretches and releases tension in the back muscles, including the muscles along the spine and in the shoulders.

- This movement can also help to improve posture by encouraging proper alignment of the spine.

- The rhythmic breathing pattern promotes relaxation and helps to calm the mind.

Caution:

- Move gently and mindfully through the Cat-Cow stretch, avoiding any jerky or forceful movements.

- If you have any pre-existing spinal or back injuries, consult with a healthcare professional before practicing this stretch.

3.5 Seated Warrior Pose

Seated Warrior Pose is a modified version of the traditional Warrior Pose (Virabhadrasana) that helps to build strength in the legs, arms, and core muscles. Here's how to practice it:

1. Sit comfortably on the edge of your chair with your feet flat on the ground and your spine tall.

2. Place your hands on your thighs or knees for support.

3. Inhale deeply as you lengthen your spine and engage your core muscles.

4. Exhale and extend your right leg out to the side, keeping your foot flat on the ground and your toes pointing forward.

5. Inhale as you raise your arms overhead, reaching towards the

ceiling with your fingertips and lengthening through your torso.

6. Exhale as you lean your upper body towards the left, keeping your right hand on your right thigh or knee for support.

7. Hold the stretch for 3-5 breaths, feeling a gentle stretch along the right side of your body.

8. Inhale to come back to center, raising your arms overhead.

9. Exhale and lower your right leg back to the starting position.

10. Repeat the stretch on the opposite side, extending your left leg out to the side and leaning your upper body towards the right.

Benefits:

- Seated Warrior Pose strengthens the legs, arms, and core muscles.

- It stretches the side body and promotes flexibility in the spine and hips.

- This pose can help to improve balance and stability.

- Seated Warrior Pose also encourages deep breathing and mindfulness, promoting relaxation and mental focus.

Caution:

- If you have knee or hip injuries, avoid extending the leg out to the side too far or putting too much weight on the extended leg.

- Listen to your body and only stretch as far as feels comfortable. If you experience any pain or discomfort, ease out of the pose and modify as needed.

CHAPTER 4

Chair Yoga Sequences

4.1 Morning Chair Yoga Routine

This chair yoga sequence is designed to help you gently awaken your body, increase energy levels, and prepare for the day ahead. Perform each pose slowly and mindfully, focusing on your breath and the sensations in your body.

1. Seated Cat-Cow Stretch:

   - Sit comfortably on the edge of your chair with your feet flat on the ground and your spine tall.

   - Place your hands on your knees or thighs.

- Inhale deeply as you arch your back and lift your chest forward (Cow pose).

- Exhale slowly as you round your spine, tucking your chin towards your chest (Cat pose).

- Repeat this movement for 6-8 breaths, moving with the rhythm of your breath.

2. Seated Twist:

- Sit tall with your feet flat on the ground and your spine elongated.

- Inhale deeply and lengthen your spine.

- Exhale as you twist your torso to the right, placing your left hand on the outside of your right knee and your right hand on the back of the chair for support.

- Hold the twist for 3-5 breaths, feeling a gentle stretch along the spine.

- Inhale to come back to center, then repeat the twist on the left side.

3. Seated Forward Bend:

   - Sit tall with your feet hip-width apart and your spine elongated.

   - Inhale deeply as you reach your arms overhead, lengthening through your torso.

   - Exhale as you hinge forward from your hips, reaching your hands towards your feet or the floor.

- Hold the stretch for 3-5 breaths, feeling a gentle stretch along the spine and the backs of the legs.

- Inhale to come back to an upright position.

4. Seated Sun Salutation:

  - Sit tall with your feet flat on the ground and your spine elongated.

  - Inhale as you sweep your arms overhead, reaching towards the ceiling.

  - Exhale as you lower your arms down to your sides.

  - Repeat this movement 3-5 times, flowing with your breath and focusing on the sensation of stretching and lengthening through your body.

5. Seated Side Stretch:

- Sit tall with your feet flat on the ground and your spine elongated.

- Inhale deeply as you raise your right arm overhead, stretching towards the left side.

- Exhale as you lean gently to the left, feeling a stretch along the right side of your body.

- Hold the stretch for 3-5 breaths, then return to an upright position and repeat on the opposite side.

6. Seated Meditation:

- Sit comfortably on the edge of your chair with your feet flat on the ground

and your hands resting on
your knees.

- Close your eyes and take
  several deep breaths,
  allowing your body and
  mind to relax.

- Bring your awareness to
  your breath, noticing the
  sensation of each inhale
  and exhale.

- Sit quietly for 5-10
  minutes, focusing on your
  breath and cultivating a
  sense of calm and
  presence.

7. Seated Neck Stretch:

- Sit tall with your feet flat
  on the ground and your
  spine elongated.

- Drop your right ear
  towards your right

shoulder, feeling a stretch along the left side of your neck.

- Hold the stretch for 3-5 breaths, then gently switch sides, dropping your left ear towards your left shoulder.

Performing this morning chair yoga routine can help you start your day with a sense of ease, vitality, and mindfulness. Customize the sequence to suit your needs and preferences, and remember to listen to your body and practice with awareness and compassion.

4.2 Relaxation Chair Yoga Sequence

This chair yoga sequence is designed to help you relax, release tension, and promote a sense of calm and well-being. Perform each pose slowly and mindfully, focusing on your breath and allowing yourself to let go of any stress or tension.

1. Seated Mountain Pose:

    - Sit comfortably on the edge of your chair with your feet flat on the ground and your spine tall.

    - Place your hands on your thighs or knees, palms facing down.

    - Close your eyes and take several deep breaths, allowing your body to relax and settle into the present moment.

    - Focus on grounding through your sit bones and lengthening through the crown of your head.

2. Seated Shoulder Rolls:

- Inhale as you lift your shoulders up towards your ears.

- Exhale as you roll your shoulders back and down, feeling a gentle stretch across the front of your chest.

- Repeat this movement 5-10 times, allowing your breath to guide the motion and release tension in your shoulders and upper back.

3. Seated Side Stretch:

- Sit tall with your feet flat on the ground and your spine elongated.

- Inhale deeply as you raise your right arm overhead, stretching towards the left side.

- Exhale as you lean gently to the left, feeling a stretch along the right side of your body.

- Hold the stretch for 3-5 breaths, then return to an upright position and repeat on the opposite side.

4. Seated Forward Bend:

- Sit tall with your feet hip-width apart and your spine elongated.

- Inhale deeply as you reach your arms overhead, lengthening through your torso.

- Exhale as you hinge forward from your hips, reaching your hands towards your feet or the floor.

- Allow your head to hang heavy and relax your neck and shoulders.

- Hold the stretch for 5-10 breaths, feeling a gentle release in your lower back and hamstrings.

5. Seated Twist:

- Sit tall with your feet flat on the ground and your spine elongated.

- Inhale deeply and lengthen your spine.

- Exhale as you twist your torso to the right, placing your left hand on the outside of your right knee and your right hand on the back of the chair for support.

- Hold the twist for 5-7 breaths, feeling a gentle twist along the spine.

- Inhale to come back to center, then repeat the twist on the left side.

6. Seated Meditation:

- Sit comfortably on the edge of your chair with your feet flat on the ground and your hands resting on your thighs.

- Close your eyes and take several deep breaths, allowing your body and mind to relax.

- Bring your awareness to your breath, noticing the sensation of each inhale and exhale.

- Allow yourself to let go of any tension or stress, and simply be present in the moment.

- Sit quietly for 5-10 minutes, allowing yourself to rest and rejuvenate.

Performing this relaxation chair yoga sequence can help you unwind, release tension, and cultivate a sense of peace and tranquility. Customize the sequence to suit your needs and preferences, and remember to listen to your body and practice with gentleness and compassion.

4.3 Chair Yoga for Stress Relief

This chair yoga sequence is specifically designed to help alleviate stress and promote relaxation. Perform each pose slowly and mindfully, focusing on your breath and allowing yourself to let go of tension and worries.

1. Seated Mountain Pose:

    - Sit comfortably on the edge of your chair with your feet flat on the ground and your spine tall.

    - Close your eyes and take several deep breaths, allowing your body to relax and settle into the present moment.

    - Place your hands on your thighs or knees, palms facing down.

    - Focus on grounding through your sit bones and lengthening through the crown of your head.

    - Hold the pose for 1-2 minutes, breathing deeply

and allowing yourself to feel supported and grounded.

2. Seated Shoulder Rolls:

   - Inhale as you lift your shoulders up towards your ears.

   - Exhale as you roll your shoulders back and down, feeling a gentle stretch across the front of your chest.

   - Repeat this movement 5-10 times, allowing your breath to guide the motion and release tension in your shoulders and upper back.

3. Seated Cat-Cow Stretch:

   - Sit tall with your feet flat on the ground and your spine elongated.

- Inhale deeply as you arch your back and lift your chest forward (Cow pose).

- Exhale slowly as you round your spine, tucking your chin towards your chest (Cat pose).

- Repeat this movement for 6-8 breaths, moving with the rhythm of your breath and allowing your spine to gently stretch and release tension.

4. Seated Forward Bend:

- Sit tall with your feet hip-width apart and your spine elongated.

- Inhale deeply as you reach your arms overhead, lengthening through your torso.

- Exhale as you hinge forward from your hips, reaching your hands towards your feet or the floor.

- Allow your head to hang heavy and relax your neck and shoulders.

- Hold the stretch for 5-10 breaths, feeling a gentle release in your lower back and hamstrings.

5. Seated Twist:

   - Sit tall with your feet flat on the ground and your spine elongated.

   - Inhale deeply and lengthen your spine.

   - Exhale as you twist your torso to the right, placing your left hand on the

outside of your right knee
and your right hand on the
back of the chair for
support.

- Hold the twist for 5-7
  breaths, feeling a gentle
  twist along the spine.

- Inhale to come back to
  center, then repeat the twist
  on the left side.

6. Seated Meditation:

- Sit comfortably on the
  edge of your chair with
  your feet flat on the ground
  and your hands resting on
  your thighs.

- Close your eyes and take
  several deep breaths,
  allowing your body and
  mind to relax.

- Bring your awareness to your breath, noticing the sensation of each inhale and exhale.

- Allow yourself to let go of any tension or stress, and simply be present in the moment.

- Sit quietly for 5-10 minutes, allowing yourself to rest and rejuvenate.

Performing this chair yoga sequence for stress relief can help you unwind, release tension, and cultivate a sense of peace and calm. Customize the sequence to suit your needs and preferences, and remember to practice with gentleness and compassion towards yourself.

CHAPTER 5

Advanced Chair Yoga Poses

5.1 Seated Eagle Pose

Seated Eagle Pose is an advanced chair yoga pose that challenges balance, coordination, and flexibility. It also helps to improve concentration and focus. Here's how to practice it:

1. Begin seated on the edge of your chair with your feet flat on the ground and your spine tall.

2. Shift your weight onto your left foot and cross your right thigh over your left thigh, bringing your right foot behind your left calf if possible. If this is too challenging, you can simply cross your right ankle over your left ankle.

3. Once your legs are crossed, press your right foot firmly against your left calf or ankle for stability.

4. Extend your arms out to the sides at shoulder height, parallel to the ground.

5. Cross your right arm under your left arm, bending your elbows and bringing your palms together if possible. If you're unable to bring your palms together, you can simply press the backs of your hands together.

6. Lift your elbows slightly and draw your shoulder blades down your back, engaging your core muscles to maintain stability.

7. Hold the pose for 3-5 breaths, maintaining a steady gaze and focusing on your breath.

8. To release, slowly unwind your arms and legs, returning to a neutral seated position.

9. Repeat the pose on the opposite side, crossing your left thigh over your right thigh and your left arm under your right arm.

Benefits:

- Seated Eagle Pose helps to improve balance, coordination, and concentration.

- It stretches the shoulders, upper back, and outer thighs.

- This pose also stimulates the muscles of the arms and legs, promoting strength and endurance.

- Seated Eagle Pose can help to relieve tension in the shoulders and upper back, reducing stiffness and promoting flexibility.

Caution:

- Avoid this pose if you have any knee or ankle injuries.

- If you experience discomfort or strain in your joints, gently release the pose and try a modified version with less intensity.

- Always listen to your body and practice within your limits, avoiding any movements that cause pain or discomfort.

5.2 Seated Pigeon Pose

Seated Pigeon Pose is an advanced chair yoga pose that provides a deep stretch to the hips and glutes. It can help alleviate tension and increase flexibility in these areas. Here's how to practice it:

1. Begin seated on the edge of your chair with your feet flat on the ground and your spine tall.

2. Plant your right foot firmly on the ground and cross your left ankle over your right thigh, just above the knee, creating a figure-four shape with your legs.

3. Flex your left foot to protect your knee and ankle joints.

4. Keep your spine tall and your chest lifted as you gently press your left knee away from your body, feeling a stretch in your left hip and glute.

5. If you'd like to deepen the stretch, gently hinge forward from your hips, keeping your back straight and your chest open.

6. Hold the pose for 3-5 deep breaths, maintaining a steady and even breath.

7. To release, slowly sit back up, uncross your legs, and return to a neutral seated position.

8. Repeat the pose on the opposite side, crossing your right ankle over your left thigh.

Benefits:

- Seated Pigeon Pose stretches the hip rotators, glutes, and piriformis muscles, helping to alleviate tension and discomfort in these areas.

- It can improve flexibility and mobility in the hips, promoting greater ease of movement.

- Seated Pigeon Pose also helps to release stress and tension stored in the hips and lower back, promoting relaxation and a sense of ease.

Caution:

- Avoid this pose if you have any knee or ankle injuries.

- If you experience discomfort or strain in your joints, gently release the pose and try a modified version with less intensity.

- Always listen to your body and practice within your limits, avoiding any movements that cause pain or discomfort.

5.3 Seated Half Lotus Pose

Seated Half Lotus Pose is an advanced chair yoga pose that provides a deep stretch to the hips and groin while also promoting relaxation and inner calm. Here's how to practice it:

1. Begin seated on the edge of your chair with your feet flat on the ground and your spine tall.

2. Bring your right foot up onto your left thigh, placing the sole of your right foot against your left thigh

as close to your hip crease as
comfortable. If this is too
challenging, you can simply bring
your right ankle to rest on your
left shin.

3. Flex your right foot to protect
    your knee joint.

4. Keep your spine tall and your
    chest lifted as you gently press
    your right knee away from your
    body, feeling a stretch in your
    right hip and groin.

5. If you'd like to deepen the stretch,
    you can gently hinge forward
    from your hips, keeping your back
    straight and your chest open.

6. Hold the pose for 3-5 deep
    breaths, maintaining a steady and
    even breath.

7. To release, slowly sit back up,
    uncross your legs, and return to a
    neutral seated position.

8. Repeat the pose on the opposite side, bringing your left foot up onto your right thigh.

Benefits:

- Seated Half Lotus Pose stretches the hips, groin, and knees, helping to increase flexibility and mobility in these areas.

- It can also help to open the hips and create space in the lower back, reducing stiffness and promoting ease of movement.

- Seated Half Lotus Pose is deeply calming and grounding, promoting relaxation and inner peace.

Caution:

- Avoid this pose if you have any knee or ankle injuries.

- If you experience discomfort or strain in your joints, gently release the pose and try a modified version with less intensity.

- Always listen to your body and practice within your limits, avoiding any movements that cause pain or discomfort.

CHAPTER 6

Chair Yoga Modifications and Props

6.1 Using Props Safely

When practicing chair yoga, props can be valuable tools to support your practice and enhance your experience. Here are some tips for using props safely:

1. Stability: Ensure that any props used provide stable support and are placed securely to prevent slipping or tipping during practice.

2. Quality: Invest in high-quality props that are durable and well-made to ensure your safety and comfort during practice.

3. Proper Placement: Position props such as blocks, straps, or blankets

within easy reach to avoid straining or overreaching during practice.

4. Listen to Your Body: Pay attention to how your body feels when using props and make adjustments as needed to ensure comfort and support. If a prop causes discomfort or pain, discontinue use or modify as necessary.

5. Consult a Professional: If you're unsure about how to use props safely or if you have specific health concerns or limitations, consider consulting a qualified yoga instructor or healthcare professional for guidance.

6.2 Modifications for Different Abilities

Chair yoga can be adapted to accommodate individuals with different abilities, mobility levels, and physical conditions. Here are some modifications to consider:

1. Seated Poses: Many traditional yoga poses can be modified to be performed while seated in a chair. For example, seated twists, forward bends, and side stretches can all be adapted for chair yoga practice.

2. Standing Poses with Support: If standing poses are included in the practice, provide support such as a chair or wall for balance and stability. For example, a standing forward bend can be practiced with the hands resting on a chair for support.

3. Gentle Movements: Focus on gentle, flowing movements that promote flexibility, mobility, and relaxation without placing strain on the body. Encourage students to move within their range of motion and avoid forcing or overstretching.

4. Breath Awareness: Incorporate breath awareness and mindfulness practices into the yoga sequence to promote relaxation and reduce stress. Encourage students to focus on their breath and cultivate a sense of inner calm and peace.

5. Personalized Guidance: Offer personalized guidance and support to students based on their individual needs and abilities. Provide options for modifications and encourage students to listen to their bodies and practice self-care.

Implementing these modifications and using props safely, chair yoga can be accessible and beneficial for individuals of all ages and abilities, providing an opportunity to experience the many benefits of yoga in a supportive and inclusive environment.

CHAPTER 7

Breathing and Meditation Techniques

7.1 Deep Breathing Exercises

Deep breathing exercises, also known as diaphragmatic or abdominal breathing, can help reduce stress, increase relaxation, and promote a sense of calm and well-being. Here are a few techniques to try:

1. Abdominal Breathing:

    - Sit comfortably in a chair with your feet flat on the ground and your hands resting on your abdomen.

    - Close your eyes and take a deep breath in through

your nose, allowing your abdomen to expand fully as you inhale.

- Exhale slowly through your mouth, letting your abdomen contract as you release the breath.

- Continue this deep breathing pattern for several breaths, focusing on the rise and fall of your abdomen with each inhale and exhale.

2. 4-7-8 Breathing:

- Sit or lie down in a comfortable position and close your eyes.

- Inhale deeply through your nose for a count of 4 seconds, filling your lungs completely with air.

- Hold your breath for a count of 7 seconds, allowing the oxygen to circulate throughout your body.

- Exhale slowly and completely through your mouth for a count of 8 seconds, releasing any tension or stress with each breath.

- Repeat this cycle of breathing for several rounds, gradually increasing the duration as you become more comfortable with the technique.

3. Box Breathing:

- Sit or stand in a comfortable position and close your eyes.

- Inhale deeply through your nose for a count of 4 seconds, imagining drawing the breath into your belly.

- Hold your breath for a count of 4 seconds, feeling the sensation of stillness and calm.

- Exhale slowly and completely through your mouth for a count of 4 seconds, releasing any tension or stress with each breath.

- Hold your breath out for a count of 4 seconds, experiencing a moment of emptiness and clarity.

- Repeat this cycle of breathing for several rounds, allowing each

breath to flow smoothly
and effortlessly.

7.2 Guided Meditation for Relaxation

Guided meditation involves following the verbal guidance of a teacher or recorded audio to lead you through a meditation practice. Here's a simple guided meditation for relaxation:

1. Find a comfortable seated position in a quiet and peaceful environment. Close your eyes and take a few deep breaths to center yourself and relax your body.

2. Bring your awareness to your breath, noticing the sensation of each inhale and exhale. Allow your breath to become slow, deep, and steady.

3. Begin to relax each part of your
    body, starting from the top of
    your head and gradually moving
    down to your toes. With each
    breath, imagine sending relaxation
    and ease to each area of your
    body, releasing any tension or
    tightness you may be holding.

4. As you continue to breathe deeply
    and relax, imagine yourself in a
    peaceful and serene place in
    nature. Picture yourself
    surrounded by beauty, tranquility,
    and gentle sounds.

5. Allow yourself to fully immerse
    in this peaceful scene, soaking up
    the sensations of calmness and
    relaxation. Stay here for a few
    moments, savoring the
    experience.

6. When you're ready, slowly bring
    your awareness back to your
    breath and your body. Take a few

more deep breaths, feeling refreshed and rejuvenated.

7. Gently open your eyes and return to the present moment, carrying the sense of relaxation and peace with you.

You can use guided meditation recordings or apps to explore different styles and themes of meditation, such as mindfulness, loving-kindness, or body scan meditations. Experiment with different techniques to find what resonates with you and helps you cultivate a greater sense of relaxation and well-being.

CHAPTER 8

Chair Yoga for Specific Conditions

8.1 Chair Yoga for Seniors

Chair yoga is an excellent option for seniors as it provides gentle movement, improves flexibility, and promotes relaxation without putting stress on the joints. Here's a chair yoga sequence tailored for seniors:

1. Seated Mountain Pose:

    - Sit tall in your chair with your feet flat on the ground, hip-width apart.

    - Rest your hands on your thighs or knees.

    - Close your eyes and take several deep breaths,

allowing your body to
relax and your mind to
become calm.

2. Seated Side Stretch:

- Inhale as you raise your
  right arm overhead.

- Exhale as you lean gently
  to the left, feeling a stretch
  along the right side of your
  body.

- Hold for a few breaths,
  then switch sides.

3. Seated Cat-Cow Stretch:

- Inhale as you arch your
  back and lift your chest
  (Cow pose).

- Exhale as you round your
  spine and tuck your chin
  (Cat pose).

- Repeat for several breaths, moving with the rhythm of your breath.

4. Seated Forward Bend:

    - Inhale as you lengthen your spine.

    - Exhale as you hinge forward from your hips, reaching your hands towards your feet or the floor.

    - Hold for a few breaths, then slowly return to an upright position.

5. Seated Twist:

    - Inhale as you lengthen your spine.

    - Exhale as you twist your torso to the right, placing your left hand on your right knee and your right hand on the back of the chair.

- Hold for a few breaths, then switch sides.

6. Ankle Rolls:

- Lift your feet off the ground and circle your ankles in one direction for a few rounds, then switch directions.

7. Wrist and Finger Stretches:

- Extend your arms out in front of you at shoulder height.

- Spread your fingers wide, then make a fist several times.

- Circle your wrists in both directions.

8. Deep Breathing:

- Close your eyes and take several deep breaths, inhaling through your nose and exhaling through your mouth.

- Focus on each inhale bringing in fresh energy and each exhale releasing tension and stress.

Chair yoga for seniors should focus on gentle movements, flexibility, and relaxation. Encourage seniors to move within their comfort level and modify poses as needed to suit their individual needs.

8.2 Chair Yoga for Office Workers

Chair yoga is an excellent way for office workers to relieve tension, reduce stress, and counteract the negative effects of prolonged sitting. Here's a chair yoga sequence tailored for office workers:

1. Seated Cat-Cow Stretch:

    - Sit tall in your chair with your feet flat on the ground.

    - Inhale as you arch your back and lift your chest (Cow pose).

    - Exhale as you round your spine and tuck your chin (Cat pose).

    - Repeat for several breaths, moving with the rhythm of your breath.

2. Seated Spinal Twist:

    - Sit tall with your feet flat on the ground.

    - Inhale as you lengthen your spine.

- Exhale as you twist your torso to the right, placing your left hand on your right knee and your right hand on the back of the chair.

- Hold for a few breaths, then switch sides.

3. Shoulder Rolls:

- Inhale as you lift your shoulders up towards your ears.

- Exhale as you roll your shoulders back and down.

- Repeat for several rounds, allowing your breath to guide the movement.

4. Neck Stretches:

- Drop your right ear towards your right shoulder, feeling a stretch along the left side of your neck.

- Hold for a few breaths, then switch sides.

- Drop your chin towards your chest, feeling a stretch along the back of your neck.

- Hold for a few breaths, then slowly lift your head back to center.

5. Wrist and Finger Stretches:

- Extend your arms out in front of you at shoulder height.

- Spread your fingers wide, then make a fist several times.

- Circle your wrists in both directions.

6. Seated Forward Fold:

- Sit tall with your feet flat on the ground.

- Inhale as you lengthen your spine.

- Exhale as you hinge forward from your hips, reaching your hands towards your feet or the floor.

- Hold for a few breaths, then slowly return to an upright position.

7. Deep Breathing:

- Close your eyes and take several deep breaths, inhaling through your nose and exhaling through your mouth.

- Focus on each inhale bringing in fresh energy

and each exhale releasing tension and stress.

Chair yoga for office workers should focus on relieving tension in the neck, shoulders, and spine, as well as promoting relaxation and stress relief. Encourage office workers to take short breaks throughout the day to practice chair yoga and relieve stiffness and fatigue associated with prolonged sitting.

CHAPTER 9

Incorporating Chair Yoga into Your Routine

Chair yoga offers a convenient and accessible way to incorporate movement, mindfulness, and relaxation into your daily routine, even if you have a busy schedule or limited mobility. Here are some tips for integrating chair yoga into your daily life:

1. Schedule Regular Practice Time:

    - Set aside dedicated time each day for chair yoga practice. This could be in the morning to start your day with relaxation and focus, during a work break to release tension and boost energy, or in the evening to unwind and prepare for sleep.

2. Start Small:

   - Begin with short chair yoga sessions, especially if you're new to yoga or have limited mobility. Even just 5-10 minutes of gentle movement and deep breathing can have significant benefits for your physical and mental well-being.

3. Be Consistent:

   - Consistency is key to experiencing the benefits of chair yoga. Aim to practice regularly, whether it's daily, several times a week, or whatever frequency works best for you. Over time, you'll

notice improvements in
your flexibility, strength,
and overall sense of well-
being.

4. Listen to Your Body:

- Pay attention to how your
  body feels during chair
  yoga practice and adjust
  your movements and
  intensity accordingly. If a
  pose or stretch feels
  uncomfortable or causes
  pain, back off or modify
  the pose to suit your needs.
  Chair yoga is all about
  meeting your body where
  it's at and practicing with
  kindness and compassion.

5. Be Mindful:

- Practice mindfulness
  during chair yoga by
  bringing your awareness to

the present moment. Focus on your breath, the sensations in your body, and the movements you're performing. Cultivate a sense of presence and awareness as you move through each pose and transition.

6. Make It Your Own:

   - Chair yoga is highly adaptable, so feel free to customize your practice to suit your preferences and needs. Experiment with different poses, breathing techniques, and meditation practices to find what feels best for you. You can also incorporate props such as blocks, straps, or blankets to enhance your practice.

7. Stay Open-Minded:

- Approach chair yoga with an open mind and a sense of curiosity. Don't be afraid to try new poses or techniques, and be willing to explore different aspects of the practice. Chair yoga offers a rich and diverse range of movements and practices that can benefit people of all ages and abilities.

8. Enjoy the Benefits:

- Finally, remember to enjoy the benefits of chair yoga! Whether it's increased flexibility, reduced stress, improved posture, or simply a greater sense of well-being, take time to appreciate how chair yoga enhances your life and overall health.

By incorporating chair yoga into your routine with these tips in mind, you can experience the transformative power of yoga in a way that's accessible, enjoyable, and sustainable for the long term.